How to beat

lung cancer

A comprehensive guide on how to survive and reverse lung cancer

Dr Micheal Wilson

Disclaimer

This book is for educational purposes only and should not be considered medical advice. It is not a substitute for professional medical care. The author and publisher are not liable for any damages or adverse effects from the use of the information provided. Consult a healthcare professional before starting any new treatment or making changes to your current treatment plan. Success is not guaranteed, and results may vary.

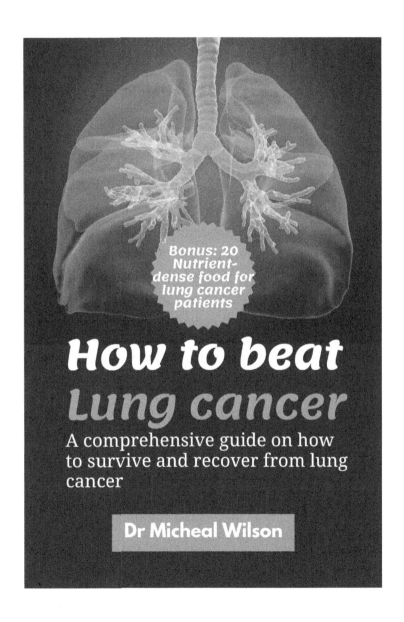

Bonus: 20 Nutrient-dense food for lung cancer patients

How to beat
Lung cancer
A comprehensive guide on how to survive and recover from lung cancer

Dr Micheal Wilson

CONTENTS

Introduction   **7**

Chapter 1: Understanding Lung Cancer   **13**

What is lung cancer?   13

Causes and risk factors   14

Types of lung cancer   16

Stages of lung cancer   19

Common symptoms and warning signs   21

Chapter 2: Diagnosis and Treatment Options   **24**

How lung cancer is diagnosed   25

Different treatment options available   27

Surgical options for lung cancer   29

Chemotherapy and radiation therapy   32

Chemotherapy and radiation therapy are two of the most commonly used treatments for lung cancer. In this part, we will discuss both treatments in detail, including how they work, their side effects, and their effectiveness in treating lung cancer.   32

Radiation Therapy for Lung Cancer Treatment 34

Effectiveness of Chemotherapy and Radiation Therapy for Lung Cancer   36

Side Effects of Chemotherapy and Radiation Therapy for Lung Cancer   38

Targeted therapy and immunotherapy   39

Challenges and Future Directions   44

Chapter 3: Coping with Diagnosis and Treatment   **46**

Emotions and feelings after a lung cancer diagnosis   46

Coping strategies for dealing with the diagnosis 49

Managing side effects of treatment   51

Importance of self-care and support system   54

Chapter 4: Nutritional Support for Recovery   58

The Significance of Proper Nutrition for Cancer Treatment and Rehabilitation   58

dietary recommendations for lung cancer patients   60

Supplements and alternative therapies   62

Chapter 5: Exercise and Physical Therapy for Recovery   70

Benefits of exercise during and after lung cancer treatment   70

Types of exercise and physical therapy for lung cancer patients   72

How to incorporate exercise into daily routine 75

Chapter 6: Managing Fatigue and Sleep Issues   80

Understanding the causes of cancer-related fatigue   80

Coping strategies for managing fatigue   83

Sleep issues and how to improve sleep quality 86

Chapter 7: Support and Resources for Lung Cancer Patients   90

Importance of support during recovery   90

Types of support and resources available for lung cancer patients 92

Finding and connecting with support groups 95

Chapter 8: Life After Lung Cancer 100

Coping with the fear of recurrence 100

Physical and emotional changes after lung cancer treatment 102

Moving forward with a new perspective on life 105

Chapter 9: Preventing Lung Cancer 108

Tips to Minimize the Chance of Developing Lung Cancer 108

Screening and early detection 110

Importance of quitting smoking 113

Bonus: 30 nutritional dense food for lung cancer patients 116

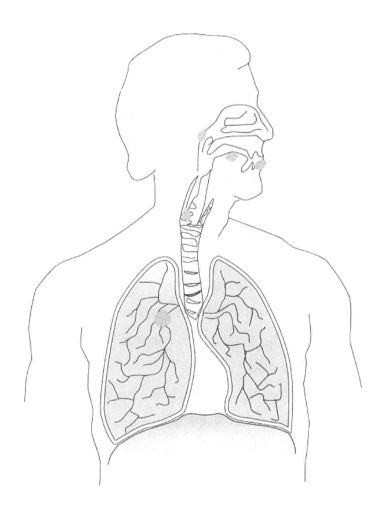

Introduction

There was this young sister of mine named Angelina who was a passionate artist, a devoted mother, and a beloved sister. However, one day, Angelina was diagnosed with lung cancer. It was a shocking and devastating moment for her and the family, and she had no idea what to do next.

Angelina had always been very close to me, her brother, and also a medical researcher. I knew about her condition and wanted to help her, but I didn't know where to start. That's when I became Angelina's guide, and I gave her a plan.

I researched extensively on different types of treatments for lung cancer and shared my knowledge with Angelina. I recommended a combination of chemotherapy and radiation therapy, which had shown promising results in patients with similar conditions.

At first, Angelina was hesitant to follow my advice, as she was worried about the side effects and the pain associated with the treatment. However, I was there to encourage her and motivate her to take action.

Angelina decided to follow my plan, and she began her treatment. It was a tough journey, but she was determined to fight cancer and emerge victorious. Despite some setbacks along the way, she continued to persevere, and with each passing day, she grew stronger and stronger. She avoided failure by staying focused on her goal and seeking support from her loved ones. Finally, after months of treatment, she got the news she had been waiting for. Her cancer was in remission! Her dedication and commitment to her treatment had paid off, and she had beaten the odds.

In the end, Angelina's story is one of courage, resilience, and determination. I played a crucial role as her guide, and my plan helped her overcome her biggest challenge. Angelina's victory over cancer was a testament to the power of love, support, and the human spirit.

The secret I want to share in this book is tested and trusted, which has helped my sister and other hundreds of people to overcome lung cancer. By the time you finish reading this book you will be convinced that lung cancer is a disease that is reversible.

Lung cancer is a devastating disease that affects millions of people worldwide. It is one of the most common types of cancer and is responsible for more deaths than any other form of cancer. While the disease is aggressive and often spreads quickly, there are many ways to recover from lung cancer and lead a healthy life once again. The journey to recovery from lung cancer is a challenging one, both physically and emotionally. But with the right mindset, support, and information, you can successfully navigate through the difficult times and come out the other side with a renewed sense of hope and purpose.

This book is a comprehensive guide on how to recover from lung cancer. It offers practical advice, real-life stories, and expert insights to help you take control of your health and well-being. Whether you are a patient, a caregiver, or someone who wants to learn more about lung cancer, this book is for you.

In the pages of this book, you will learn about the various treatments available for lung cancer, including surgery, chemotherapy, radiation therapy, and immunotherapy. You will also discover the importance of a healthy lifestyle, including exercise, nutrition, and stress management, in improving your chances of recovery.

In addition, this book covers the emotional side of lung cancer recovery. It provides strategies for coping with anxiety, depression, and other common emotional challenges that often accompany a cancer diagnosis. You will also find advice on how to communicate effectively with your loved ones, medical team, and others who can offer support during your recovery.

One of the unique aspects of this book is its focus on the power of community in healing. You will read stories from lung cancer survivors who have found strength, hope, and inspiration in connecting with others who have experienced similar struggles. You will also find resources for finding local support groups, online forums, and other communities that can offer encouragement and guidance as you navigate your recovery journey.

Throughout the book, you will encounter practical tips, exercises, and journal prompts to help you apply the information to your own life. You will also find inspiring quotes, personal stories, and insightful reflections from healthcare professionals who specialize in lung cancer treatment and recovery.

By the end of this book, you will have a comprehensive understanding of lung cancer and the steps you can take to recover from it. You will feel empowered to take control of your health and well-being, and you will have the tools you need to create a new sense of purpose and meaning in your life.

If you or someone you love has been diagnosed with lung cancer, this book is a must-read. It will give you hope, inspiration, and practical advice on how to recover from this devastating disease and live a healthy, fulfilling life once again.

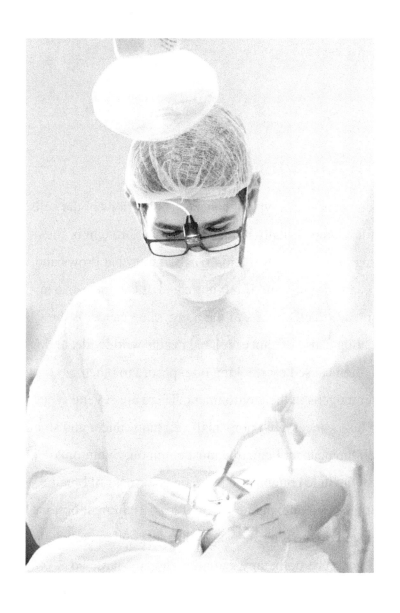

Chapter 1: Understanding Lung Cancer

What is lung cancer?

Lung cancer is a type of cancer that develops in the cells of the lungs, usually in the lining of the bronchi or the lung tissue itself. It is a malignant tumor that grows and spreads rapidly, and if left untreated, it can metastasize (spread) to other parts of the body. Lung cancer is the leading cause of cancer-related deaths worldwide, and it is often caused by smoking or exposure to other carcinogens in the environment. There are several types of lung cancer, with non-small cell lung cancer and small cell lung cancer being the most common. Symptoms may include coughing, chest pain, shortness of breath, fatigue, and unexplained weight loss. Treatment options depend on the type and stage of cancer and may include surgery, chemotherapy, radiation therapy, targeted therapy, immunotherapy, or a combination of these approaches. Early detection and treatment are important for improving outcomes and increasing the chances of survival.

Causes and risk factors

Lung cancer is a type of cancer that originates in the cells of the lung tissue. It is a serious condition that can be life-threatening. The exact cause of lung cancer is not known, but several risk factors can increase the likelihood of developing the disease. Some of the common causes and risk factors of lung cancer include:

Smoking: Smoking cigarettes, pipes, or cigars is the leading cause of lung cancer. It is estimated that smoking causes about 85% of all cases of lung cancer. Exposure to secondhand smoke: People who are regularly exposed to secondhand smoke are at an increased risk of developing lung cancer.

Radon exposure: Radon is a gas that occurs naturally and can infiltrate homes and buildings. Prolonged exposure to elevated levels of radon is known to raise the likelihood of developing lung cancer.

Occupational exposure: Exposure to certain substances in the workplace, such as asbestos, arsenic, chromium, nickel, and diesel exhaust, can increase the risk of developing lung cancer.

Air pollution: Prolonged exposure to air pollution, particularly fine particulate matter, has been linked to an increased risk of lung cancer.

Family history: A family history of lung cancer may increase the risk of developing the disease.

Personal history: People who have had lung cancer in the past are at an increased risk of developing second lung cancer.

Age: Lung cancer is a prevalent disease in individuals who are 65 years old and above.

Gender: Lung cancer is more commonly diagnosed in men than in women.

Genetics: Some genetic mutations can increase the risk of developing lung cancer.

It's important to note that not everyone who has these risk factors will develop lung cancer, and not everyone who develops lung cancer has these risk factors. However, by avoiding exposure to known risk factors and making lifestyle choices such as quitting smoking, you can reduce your risk of developing lung cancer.

Types of lung cancer

There exist two primary categories of lung cancer, namely Non-Small Cell Lung Cancer (NSCLC) and Small Cell Lung Cancer (SCLC), that are differentiated based on the visual characteristics of the cancerous cells when examined under a microscope.

Non-Small Cell Lung Cancer (NSCLC):
The most prevalent form of lung cancer is non-small cell lung cancer (NSCLC), which constitutes approximately 85% of all cases. NSCLC can be categorized into three subtypes:

Adenocarcinoma: This subtype of NSCLC starts in the cells that produce mucus and is more common in non-smokers and women. Adenocarcinoma is the most common type of lung cancer in people who have never smoked.

Squamous cell carcinoma: Squamous cell carcinoma is a variant of non-small cell lung cancer (NSCLC) that originates from the thin, flat cells that line the air passages of the lungs. Smoking is a strong risk factor for this type of cancer, and it is more frequently observed in men than in women.

Large cell carcinoma: The subtype of NSCLC known as large cell carcinoma has the potential to develop in any region of the lung and tends to exhibit rapid growth and dissemination. Typically, it is detected during an advanced stage of the disease.

Small Cell Lung Cancer (SCLC):
This particular form of lung cancer is relatively uncommon, comprising approximately 15% of all cases. SCLC is identified by small, round cancer cells that exhibit rapid growth and have a tendency to spread

aggressively to other areas of the body. It is strongly associated with smoking.

In addition to these two main types of lung cancer, other rare subtypes such as carcinoid tumors, pulmonary sarcomas, and lymphomas can also occur in the lungs. These subtypes make up less than 5% of all lung cancers.

It's important to note that these types of lung cancer can have different stages, which indicate how far cancer has spread from the initial site. The treatment and prognosis for lung cancer can vary depending on the type and stage of cancer. Surgery, chemotherapy, radiation therapy, targeted therapy, and immunotherapy are some of the treatments that may be used to manage lung cancer.

Lung cancer is often asymptomatic in the early stages, and symptoms may not appear until cancer has advanced. Therefore, it is essential to undergo regular screenings, particularly for those at high risks, such as smokers or individuals with a family history of lung cancer. Early detection and prompt treatment can improve the chances of survival and improve the quality of life for those with lung cancer.

Stages of lung cancer

The severity of lung cancer can be determined by the stage of the disease, which is based on the size and spread of the tumor.

The categorization of lung cancer into four stages is based on various factors, including the tumor's size, its position in the lung, and whether it has metastasized to other organs in the vicinity or distant parts of the body.

Stage I Lung Cancer:
In this stage, the tumor is small and localized within the lung. The tumor is usually less than 2 centimeters in size and has not spread to any other parts of the lung or nearby lymph nodes. Stage I lung cancer is often curable with surgery, which may be followed by chemotherapy or radiation therapy to kill any remaining cancer cells.

Stage II Lung Cancer:

At this phase, the tumor has enlarged and potentially metastasized to neighboring lymph nodes. It could exceed 2 centimeters or infiltrate neighboring tissues like the chest wall or diaphragm. While surgery remains a possibility, it may be combined with chemotherapy and radiation therapy to enhance the probability of a positive result.

Stage III Lung Cancer:

In this stage, the tumor has spread to lymph nodes and other tissues in the chest. The tumor may have invaded nearby organs such as the heart or esophagus, making it more difficult to treat. Treatment for Stage III lung cancer typically involves a combination of chemotherapy, radiation therapy, and surgery, depending on the location and extent of the tumor.

Stage IV Lung Cancer:

In this stage, cancer has spread to distant organs, such as the liver or brain, making it difficult to treat. Stage IV lung cancer is often considered incurable, but treatment can help to slow the growth of cancer and relieve symptoms. Treatment options for Stage IV lung cancer may include chemotherapy, targeted therapy, immunotherapy, and radiation therapy, depending on the patient's overall health and the extent of cancer.

Common symptoms and warning signs

Being aware of the common symptoms and warning signs of lung cancer can help individuals seek medical attention promptly.

Here are some common symptoms and warning signs of lung cancer:

Persistent cough: A cough that lasts for several weeks or months, particularly if it is accompanied by blood or mucus, may indicate lung cancer.

Chest pain: Lung cancer can lead to sharp chest pain that intensifies with coughing, laughing, or deep breathing.

Shortness of breath: Lung cancer may manifest as breathing difficulty or shortness of breath.

Wheezing: A high-pitched whistling sound when breathing, particularly during exhalation, may indicate lung cancer.

Fatigue: Feeling extremely tired or weak can be a symptom of lung cancer.

Weight loss: Unexplained weight loss, particularly if it is significant, can be a warning sign of lung cancer.

Loss of appetite: A decrease in appetite that persists for an extended period can be a symptom of lung cancer.

Hoarseness: Changes in voice, such as hoarseness, can be a symptom of lung cancer.

Recurrent respiratory infections: Frequent respiratory infections, such as bronchitis or pneumonia, may indicate lung cancer.

Swelling in the neck and face: Lung cancer can cause swelling in the neck and face due to the pressure exerted by a tumor on the veins leading to the heart.

Bone pain: Lung cancer that has spread to the bones can cause bone pain that may be severe.

Headaches: Lung cancer that has spread to the brain can cause headaches that are often severe and persistent.

It is crucial to acknowledge that several medical conditions can trigger some of these symptoms, and not all individuals with lung cancer will encounter these symptoms. Nevertheless, if you observe any of these indications or cautionary signs, seeking prompt medical assistance is imperative. Early recognition and management of lung cancer can increase the likelihood of successful treatment and survival.

"Hope is the only thing stronger than fear." - Robert Ludlum

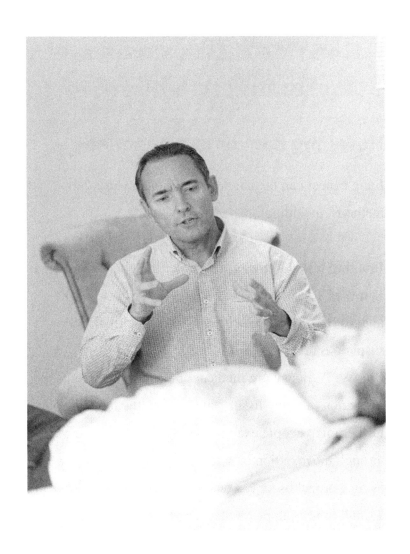

Chapter 2: Diagnosis and Treatment Options

How lung cancer is diagnosed

Lung cancer can be diagnosed through a variety of methods, including:

Imaging tests: A doctor may order imaging tests such as X-rays, CT scans, PET scans, or MRI scans to create images of the lungs and identify any abnormalities or suspicious areas.

Biopsy: A biopsy is a medical procedure that entails the extraction of a tiny tissue sample from the lungs for further microscopic examination. This can be achieved through the insertion of a needle through the skin or by using a bronchoscopy, a technique that involves inserting a small tube equipped with a camera through the nose or mouth and into the lungs.

Sputum cytology: Sputum cytology is a diagnostic procedure that examines a specimen of phlegm expectorated from the respiratory tract to detect the presence of cancerous cells.

Blood tests: Blood tests can check for markers that may be associated with lung cancer, such as tumor-specific antigens.

Lung function tests: These tests measure how well the lungs are working and can help identify any lung problems that may be related to cancer.

Clinical examination: A doctor may also perform a physical exam to check for any signs or symptoms of lung cancer, such as a persistent cough, shortness of breath, or chest pain.

It's important to note that a combination of these methods may be used to diagnose lung cancer, and the exact approach will depend on the individual case and the recommendations of the treating physician. Early diagnosis and treatment are crucial in improving the outcomes for patients with lung cancer.

Different treatment options available

The treatment options available for lung cancer depend on several factors, including the stage of cancer, the type of lung cancer, the patient's overall health, and the patient's preferences.

Here are the different treatment options available for lung cancer:

Surgery: Surgery is frequently the initial treatment option for early-stage lung cancer. The primary objective of surgery is to excise the cancerous tissue along with some adjacent healthy tissue to ensure the complete eradication of cancer cells. The type of surgical procedure selected depends on the size and location of the tumor. Partial lung removal may be necessary in some cases, while in others, the whole lung may require removal.

Radiation Therapy: Radiation Therapy is a cancer treatment that utilizes high-energy radiation to eliminate cancerous cells. Typically, it is employed for treating the initial stages of lung cancer or in combination with other therapies for advanced-stage lung cancer. Two types of radiation therapy exist, namely external beam radiation therapy and internal radiation therapy, also known as brachytherapy.

Chemotherapy: Chemotherapy is a medical procedure that involves the use of drugs to eliminate cancer cells. It is frequently employed for advanced lung cancer or as an adjunct to surgery or radiation therapy. Administration of chemotherapy drugs can be through intravenous injection or oral ingestion.

Targeted Therapy: Targeted therapy is a treatment that targets specific molecules or proteins that are involved in the growth and spread of cancer cells. This treatment is often used for advanced-stage lung cancer or as a complementary treatment to chemotherapy.

Immunotherapy: Immunotherapy is a treatment that uses the patient's own immune system to fight cancer. This treatment is often used for advanced-stage lung cancer or as a complementary treatment to chemotherapy or radiation therapy.

Palliative Care: Palliative care is specialized medical care that focuses on relieving symptoms and improving the quality of life for patients with serious illnesses, including lung cancer. Palliative care can be used at any stage of the disease and can be used in combination with other treatments.

It is important to note that the treatment plan for lung cancer may involve a combination of these treatment options. The treatment plan will be tailored to the individual patient's needs, and the goal of treatment is to provide the best possible outcome while minimizing side effects. It is important for patients to discuss the available treatment options with their healthcare team to make informed decisions about their care.

Surgical options for lung cancer

The treatment of localized or early-stage lung cancer often involves surgical interventions, which offer a potential cure for certain patients. Nevertheless, not all patients may qualify for surgery, and the recommended surgical approach is dependent on several factors such as cancer's stage, tumor size and location, and the patient's general health.

Here are some of the surgical options for lung cancer:

Lobectomy: This is the most common surgical procedure for lung cancer, and it involves removing the entire lobe of the lung that contains the tumor. This surgery is usually recommended for patients with early-stage lung cancer, and it can be performed using traditional open surgery or minimally invasive techniques such as video-assisted thoracic surgery (VATS).

Segmentectomy: This surgery involves removing a segment of the lung that contains the tumor, instead of the entire lobe. This surgery is usually recommended for patients with small tumors or tumors that are located in a specific part of the lung, and it can also be performed using open surgery or minimally invasive techniques.

Wedge resection: This surgery involves removing a small wedge-shaped piece of the lung that contains the tumor. This surgery is usually recommended for patients with very small tumors or tumors that are located near the edge of the lung, and it can also be performed using open surgery or minimally invasive techniques.

Pneumonectomy: This surgery involves removing the entire lung that contains the tumor. This surgery is usually recommended for patients with larger tumors or tumors that are located in a specific part of the lung, and it is usually performed using open surgery.

Sleeve resection: This surgery involves removing a portion of the bronchus (the airway that leads to the lung) that contains the tumor, and then reconnecting the remaining bronchus to the lung. This surgery is usually recommended for patients with tumors that are located in the center of the lung, and it can be performed using open surgery or minimally invasive techniques.

Mediastinal lymph node dissection: This is a procedure that is usually performed in conjunction with lung cancer surgery, and it involves removing lymph nodes from the mediastinum (the area between the lungs). This procedure is important for determining the stage of cancer and for preventing the spread of cancer to other parts of the body.

It is important to note that not all patients with lung cancer are eligible for surgery. Patients with advanced-stage lung cancer, or those who have other medical conditions that make surgery too risky, may not be good candidates for surgery. In such cases, other treatments such as radiation therapy, chemotherapy, or targeted therapy may be recommended.

Chemotherapy and radiation therapy

Chemotherapy and radiation therapy are two of the most commonly used treatments for lung cancer. In this part, we will discuss both treatments in detail, including how they work, their side effects, and their effectiveness in treating lung cancer.

Chemotherapy for Lung Cancer Treatment

Chemotherapy refers to a cancer treatment that employs drugs to eliminate cancer cells. These drugs can be administered through different methods, such as orally, intravenously, or topically. Chemotherapy drugs specifically target rapidly dividing cells, which encompasses cancer cells and other healthy cells in the body, including those in the digestive tract, bone marrow, and hair follicles. As a result, chemotherapy can lead to several side effects.

Chemotherapy can be used as the primary treatment for lung cancer or as an adjunct to surgery or radiation therapy. In some cases, it can also be used to relieve symptoms caused by lung cancer, such as pain, shortness of breath, and coughing.

The most common chemotherapy drugs used for lung cancer are cisplatin, carboplatin, etoposide, and paclitaxel. These drugs are often given in combination, as this has been shown to be more effective than using a single drug.

The side effects of chemotherapy depend on the drugs used, the dose, and the individual's overall health. Common side effects include nausea and vomiting, fatigue, hair loss, mouth sores, and an increased risk of infection. Most side effects are temporary and can be managed with medications and supportive care.

Radiation Therapy for Lung Cancer Treatment

Radiation therapy is a frequently utilized approach in the treatment of lung cancer. This treatment modality employs high-energy radiation, such as X-rays or protons, to eliminate cancerous cells. The administration of radiation therapy can take place externally via a machine that directs radiation at the tumor from outside the body, or internally, via radioactive materials positioned directly within the tumor or adjacent tissue. Radiation therapy can be used as the primary treatment for lung cancer, especially in cases where surgery is not an option. It can also be used before or after surgery to shrink the tumor or kill any remaining cancer cells. In addition, radiation therapy can be used to relieve symptoms caused by lung cancer, such as pain and difficulty breathing.

The impact of radiation therapy's adverse effects varies based on the amount and location of the body being treated. Among the typical consequences are exhaustion, skin alterations, and inflammation of the lungs and esophagus. Certain individuals may also encounter challenges in swallowing, nausea, and vomiting. Fortunately, these effects are generally short-term and can be relieved with medical assistance and supportive measures.

Combining Chemotherapy and Radiation Therapy

In some cases, chemotherapy and radiation therapy may be used together to treat lung cancer. This is known as concurrent chemoradiation. The goal of this treatment is to enhance the effectiveness of radiation therapy by making cancer cells more sensitive to radiation.

The combination of chemotherapy and radiation therapy can be more effective than either treatment alone. However, it can also increase the side effects of both treatments. Common side effects of concurrent chemoradiation include fatigue, nausea, vomiting, and a decreased white blood cell count.

Effectiveness of Chemotherapy and Radiation Therapy for Lung Cancer

The effectiveness of chemotherapy and radiation therapy for lung cancer depends on several factors, including the type and stage of cancer, the patient's overall health, and the treatment plan used.

Chemotherapy has been shown to improve survival rates in patients with advanced lung cancer. A study published in the New England Journal of Medicine found that adding chemotherapy to radiation therapy increased the five-year survival rate of patients with stage III non-small cell lung cancer from 16% to 23%. Another study published in the Lancet Oncology found that combining chemotherapy with immunotherapy led to better overall survival and progression-free survival than chemotherapy alone in patients with advanced non-small cell lung cancer.

Radiation therapy is also effective in treating lung cancer, especially when used in combination with other treatments. A study published in the Journal of Thoracic

Oncology found that patients with stage III non-small cell lung cancer who received concurrent chemoradiation had a higher two-year survival rate than those who received sequential chemoradiation or radiation therapy alone.

In addition, new advancements in radiation therapy, such as stereotactic body radiation therapy (SBRT), have shown promising results in treating early-stage lung cancer. SBRT is a highly precise form of radiation therapy that delivers high doses of radiation to the tumor while minimizing exposure to surrounding healthy tissue.

Side Effects of Chemotherapy and Radiation Therapy for Lung Cancer

Both chemotherapy and radiation therapy can have side effects that can affect the patient's quality of life.

Common side effects of chemotherapy include:

Nausea and vomiting

Fatigue

Hair loss

Mouth sores

Increased risk of infection

Diarrhea or constipation

Peripheral neuropathy (numbness or tingling in the hands and feet)

Anemia (low red blood cell count)

Thrombocytopenia (low platelet count)

Common side effects of radiation therapy include:

Fatigue

Skin changes (redness, dryness, itching, or blistering)

Inflammation of the lungs or esophagus

Difficulty swallowing

Nausea and vomiting

Diarrhea

Bladder or bowel changes

Lymphedema (swelling in the arms or legs)

Targeted therapy and immunotherapy

In recent years, there has been a growing interest in targeted therapy and immunotherapy as new approaches for the treatment of lung cancer. This section will provide a comprehensive overview of these two treatment modalities and their potential use in the management of lung cancer.

Targeted Therapy for Lung Cancer Treatment

Targeted therapy is a treatment approach that involves the use of drugs that are designed to target specific molecules or pathways that are involved in the development and progression of cancer. Unlike traditional chemotherapy, which can affect both cancerous and healthy cells, targeted therapy is designed to specifically target cancer cells, while minimizing damage to healthy cells. Targeted therapy has been used to treat several types of cancer, including lung cancer.

One of the most well-known targeted therapies for lung cancer is the use of tyrosine kinase inhibitors (TKIs). TKIs work by blocking the activity of specific proteins called tyrosine kinases, which are involved in the growth and survival of cancer cells. In non-small cell lung cancer (NSCLC), mutations in the epidermal growth factor receptor (EGFR) gene are common, and several TKIs have been developed to specifically target these mutations. Examples of these drugs include erlotinib, gefitinib, and afatinib. TKIs have been shown to improve overall survival in patients with NSCLC harboring EGFR mutations, with response rates of up to 70%.

Another targeted therapy option for NSCLC is the use of anaplastic lymphoma kinase (ALK) inhibitors. In a small subset of NSCLC patients, the ALK gene is mutated, leading to the overexpression of the ALK protein. Drugs such as crizotinib, ceritinib, and alectinib have been developed to specifically target this mutation. Clinical trials have shown that these drugs can lead to significant improvements in progression-free survival and overall survival in patients with ALK-positive NSCLC.

Immunotherapy for Lung Cancer Treatment

Immunotherapy is a treatment approach that involves the use of drugs that help the patient's immune system recognize and attack cancer cells. Cancer cells can often evade the immune system by expressing proteins that inhibit the immune response, or by changing their surface proteins to make them less recognizable to immune cells. Immunotherapy drugs work by blocking these proteins or by activating immune cells to recognize and attack cancer cells.

One type of immunotherapy that has shown promise in the treatment of lung cancer is immune checkpoint inhibitors. Immune checkpoint inhibitors work by blocking proteins on the surface of T cells, such as CTLA-4 and PD-1, which normally act to inhibit the immune response. By blocking these proteins, immune checkpoint inhibitors allow the immune system to recognize and attack cancer cells. Examples of immune checkpoint inhibitors used in lung cancer treatment include nivolumab, pembrolizumab, and atezolizumab.

Clinical trials have shown that immune checkpoint inhibitors can lead to significant improvements in overall survival and progression-free survival in patients with advanced NSCLC. In fact, some studies have shown that immune checkpoint inhibitors can be more effective than traditional chemotherapy in certain patient populations. For example, in patients with advanced NSCLC whose tumors express high levels of PD-L1, pembrolizumab has been shown to be more effective than chemotherapy, with improved response rates and longer overall survival.

Combination Therapy

While targeted therapy and immunotherapy are both promising treatment approaches for lung cancer, they each have their limitations. For example, not all patients with lung cancer will have mutations that are targeted to specific drugs, and not all patients will respond to immunotherapy. In recent years, there has been growing interest in combining targeted therapy and immunotherapy to improve treatment outcomes for patients with lung cancer.

One example of combination therapy is the use of immune checkpoint inhibitors with chemotherapy. Chemotherapy drugs can help to activate the immune system by causing cancer cells to release proteins that can be recognized by immune cells. When combined with immune checkpoint inhibitors, chemotherapy can help to enhance the immune response and improve treatment outcomes in patients with advanced NSCLC. Clinical trials have shown that the combination of pembrolizumab and chemotherapy can lead to significant improvements in overall survival and progression-free survival in patients with advanced NSCLC, regardless of PD-L1 expression levels.

Another example of combination therapy is the use of targeted therapy and immunotherapy. Preclinical studies have shown that the combination of TKIs and immune checkpoint inhibitors can lead to improved treatment outcomes in patients with NSCLC. Clinical trials are currently underway to evaluate the efficacy of this approach.

Challenges and Future Directions

While targeted therapy and immunotherapy have shown promise in the treatment of lung cancer, there are still challenges to overcome. One major challenge is the development of resistance to these treatments. Cancer cells can evolve and adapt to treatment, leading to the development of resistance and the eventual failure of therapy. Researchers are working to better understand the mechanisms of resistance and to develop strategies to overcome it.

Another challenge is identifying the patients who are most likely to benefit from these treatments. While biomarkers like EGFR mutations and PD-L1 expression can help to predict response to targeted therapy and immunotherapy, not all patients with these biomarkers will respond to treatment. Researchers are working to develop new biomarkers that can better predict treatment response and improve patient selection.

In addition, there is a need for new and improved treatments for patients with lung cancer who do not respond to current therapies. Researchers are exploring new targeted therapy and immunotherapy approaches, as well as other treatment modalities like cancer vaccines and adoptive T-cell therapy.

"Believe you can and you're halfway there." - Theodore Roosevelt

Chapter 3: Coping with Diagnosis and Treatment

Emotions and feelings after a lung cancer diagnosis

Being diagnosed with lung cancer is a life-altering experience that can trigger a wide range of emotions and feelings. For many individuals, it is a traumatic experience that can leave them feeling overwhelmed, anxious, and depressed. Coping with a lung cancer diagnosis requires an understanding of the emotions and feelings that may arise during this difficult time.

Shock and disbelief are common emotions that individuals experience upon receiving a lung cancer diagnosis. It may take some time to fully comprehend the diagnosis and the impact it will have on one's life. The shock may be accompanied by a sense of disbelief or denial, which can be a normal coping mechanism to help one come to terms with the diagnosis.

Fear and anxiety are also common emotional responses to a lung cancer diagnosis. The fear of the unknown, the fear of pain, and the fear of death can all contribute to feelings of anxiety. The uncertainty surrounding the treatment process and the prognosis can also exacerbate anxiety levels.

Sadness and grief are also common emotions experienced after a lung cancer diagnosis. It is not uncommon for individuals to experience a sense of loss, even if they have not yet begun treatment. They may grieve the loss of their health, their lifestyle, and their independence. This grief may continue throughout the treatment process, as individuals may experience physical and emotional changes that further impact their sense of loss.

Anger and frustration may also be common emotions experienced after a lung cancer diagnosis. Individuals may feel angry at the situation, angry at themselves, or angry at others. They may feel frustrated with the healthcare system, with their treatment options, or with their own limitations.

Depression is also a common emotional response to a lung cancer diagnosis. Individuals may experience a sense of hopelessness, a lack of energy, and a loss of interest in activities that were once enjoyable. They may withdraw from social situations and feel isolated and alone.

Finally, hope and resilience are also important emotions that can be experienced after a lung cancer diagnosis. Individuals may find hope in their treatment options, in the support of loved ones, or in their own resilience. They may find strength in their ability to face this challenge and emerge on the other side.

Coping strategies for dealing with the diagnosis

Being diagnosed with lung cancer can be a challenging and overwhelming experience for individuals and their loved ones. It is normal to feel a range of emotions such as fear, sadness, anger, and anxiety. Coping strategies are essential in managing the emotional and physical effects of the diagnosis, as well as in making informed decisions about treatment options. Here are some coping strategies that may be helpful in dealing with the diagnosis of lung cancer:

Seek Support from Loved Ones: The support of family and friends can be invaluable during this time. Share your feelings with them, and allow them to provide you with emotional support. They can also help with practical tasks such as running errands, cooking, and cleaning.

Join a Support Group: Joining a support group can provide a safe space to discuss your experiences with people who are going through similar challenges. This can be an opportunity to share coping strategies, learn from others, and provide mutual support.

Seek Professional Support: Consider seeking professional help from a counselor, social worker, or psychologist. They can help you cope with the emotional stress of the diagnosis and provide you with tools to manage anxiety and depression.

Educate Yourself: Learning about lung cancer can help you make informed decisions about your treatment options. Speak to your healthcare provider, and do your own research on the disease and its treatments.

Practice Self-Care: Taking care of yourself is essential during this time. This can involve engaging in activities that you enjoy, such as reading, gardening, or listening to music. It can also involve taking care of your physical health by eating a healthy diet, getting enough sleep, and exercising.

Consider Complementary Therapies: Some people find complementary therapies such as acupuncture, massage, or meditation helpful in managing the physical and emotional effects of lung cancer. Speak to your healthcare provider before trying any new therapy.

Maintain a Positive Outlook: Maintaining a positive outlook can be challenging, but it can help you cope with the challenges of lung cancer. Try to focus on the positive aspects of your life, and practice gratitude for the things you are thankful for.

Managing side effects of treatment

The treatment of lung cancer often involves a combination of surgery, radiation therapy, chemotherapy, targeted therapy, and immunotherapy. While these treatments can be effective in shrinking or eliminating cancer cells, they can also cause side effects that can impact a patient's quality of life. Here are some ways to manage the side effects of lung cancer treatment:

Nausea and vomiting: Nausea and vomiting are typical outcomes of chemotherapy and radiation therapy, which can be managed by utilizing anti-nausea medications, such as ondansetron or Aprepitant. Additionally, making dietary adjustments like consuming small, frequent meals and avoiding fatty or spicy foods can aid in lessening these symptoms.

Fatigue: Fatigue is a common side effect of cancer treatment and can be caused by both cancer itself and the treatment. Getting enough rest, eating a healthy diet, and staying hydrated can help combat fatigue. It is also important to engage in light physical activity, such as walking or yoga, to maintain strength and energy.

Hair loss: Chemotherapy can cause hair loss, which can be distressing for many patients. Wearing a wig or headscarf can help conceal hair loss, and gentle hair care, such as using a mild shampoo and avoiding hot styling tools, can help promote healthy hair regrowth after treatment.

Skin changes: Radiation therapy can cause skin changes, such as redness, dryness, and itching, in the treated area. Moisturizing the skin regularly, avoiding hot water and harsh soaps, and wearing loose-fitting clothing can help reduce skin irritation.

Mouth sores: Chemotherapy can cause mouth sores, which can make eating and speaking difficult. Using a soft-bristled toothbrush, avoiding spicy or acidic foods, and rinsing the mouth with salt water or baking soda solution can help soothe mouth sores.

Loss of appetite: Cancer treatment can cause a loss of appetite, which can lead to weight loss and malnutrition. Eating small, frequent meals and snacks, choosing high-calorie, high-protein foods, and drinking fluids between meals can help maintain adequate nutrition.

Cognitive changes: Cancer treatment can cause cognitive changes, such as difficulty concentrating or memory loss, which can impact daily activities. Engaging in mentally stimulating activities, such as reading or doing puzzles, and getting enough rest can help improve cognitive function.

Emotional side effects: Cancer treatment can also cause emotional side effects, such as anxiety, depression, and mood swings. Talking to a therapist or counselor, participating in support groups, and practicing relaxation techniques, such as deep breathing or meditation, can help manage these symptoms.

Importance of self-care and support system

Lung cancer is a devastating illness that can have a significant impact on a person's life. Managing the disease requires a comprehensive approach that includes both medical and emotional support. Self-care and a strong support system can help individuals with lung cancer cope with the challenges of the disease and maintain a good quality of life.

It is essential for people with lung cancer to prioritize self-care, which encompasses taking care of one's physical, emotional, and mental well-being. Physical self-care entails maintaining a healthy diet, engaging in regular exercise, and ensuring adequate sleep. Fatigue is a common issue among individuals with lung cancer, and physical activity and rest can help alleviate this symptom.

Emotional self-care involves recognizing and managing one's emotions. A cancer diagnosis can be emotionally overwhelming, and individuals may experience anxiety, depression, or fear. It's essential to seek professional help to address these emotions and develop coping strategies.

Mental self-care involves stimulating the mind and engaging in activities that promote well-being. Individuals with lung cancer may experience brain fog or memory problems due to the disease or treatment. Engaging in activities such as reading, crossword puzzles, or other mentally stimulating tasks can help combat these issues.

A strong support system is also essential for individuals with lung cancer. A support system can provide emotional support, practical assistance, and social connections. This system can consist of family, friends, healthcare providers, or support groups. The support system should be non-judgmental, and understanding, and provide a safe space to express feelings.

Having a strong support system can help individuals with lung cancer manage the stress of the disease and treatment. Family members or friends can provide practical support such as transportation to appointments, help with household chores, or childcare. Support groups can provide a sense of community and understanding among individuals who are going through similar experiences.

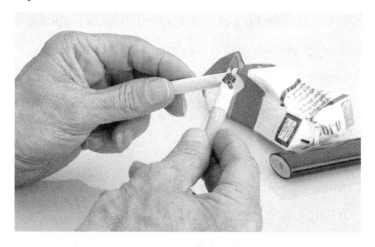

"Strength does not come from physical capacity. It comes from an indomitable will." - Mahatma Gandhi

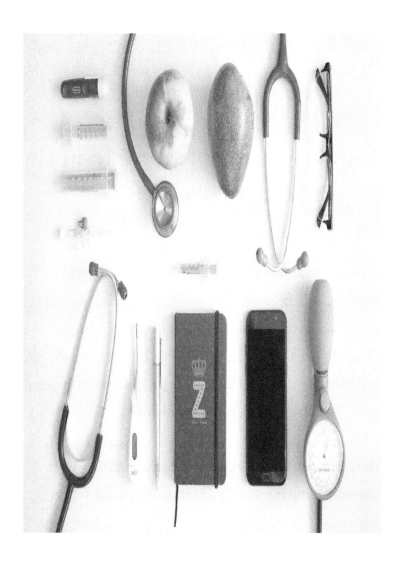

Chapter 4: Nutritional Support for Recovery

The Significance of Proper Nutrition for Cancer Treatment and Rehabilitation

Nutrition plays a crucial role in the treatment and recovery of cancer patients. The body requires energy and nutrients to fight off cancer cells and recover from the side effects of cancer treatments. Eating a healthy and balanced diet can help cancer patients maintain their strength, energy levels, and overall health.

Here are some of the ways in which nutrition is important during cancer treatment and recovery:

Boosting the immune system: A strong immune system is essential for fighting off cancer cells and preventing infections. Eating a diet rich in fruits, vegetables, whole grains, lean proteins, and healthy fats can help boost the immune system and provide the body with the nutrients it needs to function properly.

Reducing side effects of treatment: Cancer treatments such as chemotherapy and radiation therapy can cause side effects like nausea, vomiting, and diarrhea. Eating small, frequent meals throughout the day, staying hydrated, and avoiding spicy or greasy foods can help reduce these side effects and make treatment more tolerable.

Preventing malnutrition: Cancer and cancer treatments can lead to weight loss, muscle wasting, and malnutrition. Eating a balanced diet that includes protein, carbohydrates, and healthy fats can help prevent malnutrition and maintain a healthy weight.

Promoting healing: Surgery, radiation therapy, and chemotherapy can all cause tissue damage and inflammation. Eating a diet rich in antioxidants, vitamins, and minerals can help promote healing and reduce inflammation.

Improving the quality of life: Cancer and cancer treatments can take a toll on a patient's physical and emotional well-being. Eating a healthy and balanced diet can help improve mood, energy levels, and overall quality of life.

Reducing the risk of cancer recurrence: Eating a healthy diet and maintaining a healthy weight can help reduce the risk of cancer recurrence. Studies have shown that a diet rich in fruits, vegetables, whole grains, and lean proteins can help prevent cancer recurrence.

dietary recommendations for lung cancer patients

Individuals diagnosed with lung cancer often require dietary modifications that are distinct from those of healthy individuals. A nutritious and well-rounded diet can play a crucial role in fortifying the immune system, diminishing inflammation, and promoting general health and wellness. The following are some dietary guidelines that may benefit lung cancer patients:

Consume a diet high in fruits and vegetables: Fruits and vegetables are high in vitamins, minerals, and antioxidants, which can help protect the body against the harmful effects of free radicals. Choose a variety of colorful fruits and vegetables such as spinach, carrots, berries, and citrus fruits.

Incorporate lean protein sources: Protein is a vital nutrient for constructing and mending tissues. Opt for lean protein sources, such as eggs, fish, chicken, turkey, beans, and legumes.

Avoid processed and red meats: Processed and red meats have been linked to an increased risk of cancer. Limit your intake of bacon, sausage, hot dogs, and beef.

Opt for whole grains: Whole grains are an excellent source of fiber, which can aid in the regulation of digestion and the reduction of inflammation. Opt for whole-grain bread, pasta, and rice.

Reduce intake of saturated and trans fats: Saturated and trans fats can increase inflammation in the body. Limit your intake of butter, cream, and fried foods.

Drink plenty of fluids: Ensuring proper hydration is crucial for maintaining good health. Consume ample amounts of water, herbal tea, and other beverages that are not high in sugar content.

Consider supplementation: Certain supplements may help support the immune system and reduce inflammation. Speak to your healthcare provider about supplements such as vitamin D, omega-3 fatty acids, and probiotics.

Avoid alcohol and tobacco: Alcohol and tobacco can increase inflammation in the body and increase the risk of cancer. Avoid alcohol and tobacco products.

Consult with a registered dietitian: A registered dietitian can help you develop a personalized nutrition plan that meets your specific needs and preferences.

Supplements and alternative therapies

There are various options available for treating lung cancer, which includes surgery, chemotherapy, radiation therapy, and targeted therapy. However, some people also use supplements and alternative therapies in addition to traditional treatments to manage symptoms or improve their overall well-being. Let's explore some of the supplements and alternative therapies that are commonly used for lung cancer.

Supplements:

Vitamin D:

Vitamin D is a nutrient that is essential for maintaining healthy bones, teeth, and muscles. Recent studies suggest that vitamin D may also play a role in preventing or treating lung cancer. Research has shown that people with low levels of vitamin D in their blood are at a higher risk of developing lung cancer. Additionally, studies have shown that vitamin D may help in reducing the growth and spread of cancer cells. Therefore, vitamin D supplements may be beneficial for lung cancer patients, especially those with low levels of vitamin D in their blood.

Omega-3 fatty acids:

Omega-3 fatty acids are essential fats that play a crucial role in maintaining good health. Studies have suggested that omega-3 fatty acids may help in reducing inflammation, which is a major risk factor for developing cancer. Additionally, studies have also shown that omega-3 fatty acids may help in improving the effectiveness of chemotherapy drugs. Therefore, omega-3 fatty acid supplements may be helpful for lung cancer patients.

Melatonin:

The pineal gland in the brain synthesizes a hormone called melatonin. It helps in regulating the sleep-wake cycle and may also have anti-cancer properties. Studies have suggested that melatonin may help in reducing the growth and spread of cancer cells. Additionally, melatonin may also help in reducing the side effects of chemotherapy and radiation therapy. Therefore, melatonin supplements may be beneficial for lung cancer patients.

Vitamin C:

Vitamin C is a nutrient that is essential for maintaining good health. Studies have suggested that vitamin C may help in reducing the risk of developing lung cancer. Additionally, vitamin C may also help in reducing the side effects of chemotherapy and radiation therapy. Therefore, vitamin C supplements may be helpful for lung cancer patients.

Alternative Therapies:

Acupuncture:

Acupuncture, a traditional healing method from China, entails the insertion of fine needles into particular body points. Its purpose is to restore energy balance within the body and alleviate symptoms linked to cancer, including pain. Research indicates that acupuncture may aid in minimizing the adverse effects of chemotherapy and radiation therapy, making it a potentially beneficial therapy for individuals with lung cancer.

Yoga:

Yoga is an ancient Indian practice that involves physical postures, breathing exercises, and meditation. It is believed to help in reducing stress and anxiety, which are common among cancer patients. Additionally, studies have suggested that yoga may also help in reducing the side effects of chemotherapy and radiation therapy. Therefore, yoga may be helpful for lung cancer patients.

Massage therapy:

Massage therapy involves manipulating the soft tissues of the body, such as muscles and tendons, to promote relaxation and relieve pain. Studies have suggested that massage therapy may help in reducing pain, anxiety, and depression in cancer patients. Therefore, massage therapy may be helpful for lung cancer patients.

Mind-body techniques:

Mind-body techniques, such as meditation and guided imagery, involve using the power of the mind to promote healing and reduce stress. Studies have suggested that these techniques may help in reducing the side effects of chemotherapy and radiation therapy. Therefore, mind-body techniques may be helpful for lung cancer patients.

It is important to note that supplements and alternative therapies should not be used as a replacement for traditional medical treatments for lung cancer. These approaches should only be used as complementary therapy under the guidance of a healthcare professional. It is also important to consider potential risks and side effects associated with supplements and alternative therapies.

It's crucial to be aware that supplements, including those labeled as natural, may have adverse side effects or interact negatively with medications when consumed in excessive amounts. For instance, high doses of vitamin C can obstruct the effectiveness of chemotherapy and radiation therapy, while melatonin may clash with blood-thinning medications. Therefore, seeking guidance from a healthcare expert before initiating any supplement routine is highly recommended.

Similarly, alternative therapies such as acupuncture and massage therapy may not be suitable for everyone. People with certain medical conditions or those taking blood-thinning medications should avoid acupuncture. Massage therapy can cause bruising or bleeding in people with low platelet counts, which is a common side effect of chemotherapy. It is important to discuss alternative therapy options with a healthcare professional to ensure they are safe and effective for each individual case.

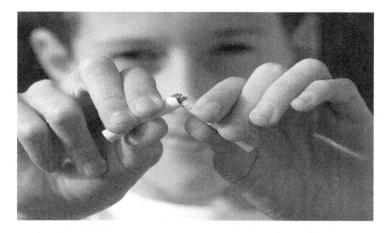

"The greatest glory in living lies not in never falling, but in rising every time we fall." - Nelson Mandela

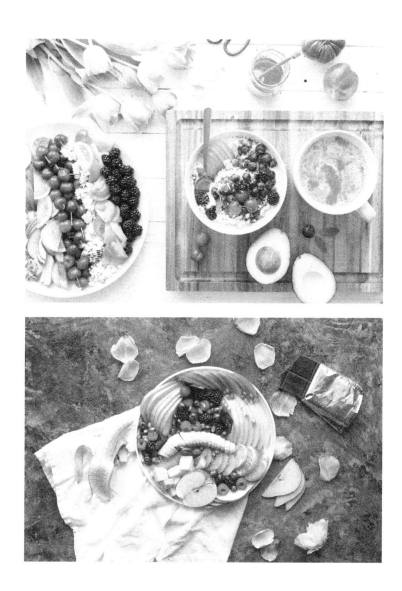

Chapter 5: Exercise and Physical Therapy for Recovery

Benefits of exercise during and after lung cancer treatment

Exercise has been shown to have many benefits during and after lung cancer treatment, including:

Improved respiratory function: Exercise can help improve respiratory function by strengthening the muscles involved in breathing. This can help improve lung capacity and reduce shortness of breath, which is a common side effect of lung cancer treatment.

Reduced fatigue: Fatigue is a common side effect of lung cancer treatment, but exercise has been shown to help reduce fatigue and improve energy levels. This can help improve quality of life during treatment and beyond.

Improved mood: Exercise has been shown to have a positive effect on mood and mental health. This can be particularly beneficial for lung cancer patients who may experience anxiety, depression, or other emotional challenges during treatment.

Increased muscle strength: Lung cancer treatment can cause muscle weakness and loss of muscle mass, but exercise can help increase muscle strength and preserve muscle mass.

Reduced risk of recurrence: Regular exercise has been shown to reduce the risk of cancer recurrence and improve overall survival in cancer patients.

Improved cardiovascular health: Exercise can help improve cardiovascular health by reducing blood pressure, improving circulation, and reducing the risk of heart disease. This can be particularly important for lung cancer patients who may have an increased risk of cardiovascular complications.

Improved bone health: Lung cancer treatment can increase the risk of bone loss and fractures, but exercise can help improve bone health and reduce the risk of osteoporosis.

Improved immune function: Exercise has been shown to have a positive effect on immune function, which can help improve overall health and reduce the risk of infection.

Improved quality of life: Exercise can help improve overall quality of life by reducing symptoms and side effects of treatment, improving mood and energy levels, and increasing physical function.

Types of exercise and physical therapy for lung cancer patients

Lung cancer patients may experience physical limitations due to the effects of cancer and its treatments, which can include surgery, chemotherapy, and radiation therapy. Exercise and physical therapy are important components of a comprehensive cancer care plan and can help improve physical function, quality of life, and overall well-being.

There are several types of exercises and physical therapy interventions that may be beneficial for lung cancer patients. These include:

Aerobic exercise: Aerobic exercise involves activities that increase heart rate and breathing, such as walking, cycling, swimming, or dancing. These activities can help improve cardiovascular function, increase endurance, and enhance overall fitness. Aerobic exercise can also help reduce fatigue and improve mood and emotional well-being.

Resistance training: Resistance training involves the use of weights, resistance bands, or body weight exercises to build strength and improve muscle tone. This type of exercise can help prevent muscle loss and improve functional capacity, making it easier for lung cancer patients to perform activities of daily living. Resistance training is a beneficial way to enhance bone density and decrease the likelihood of osteoporosis.

Breathing exercises: Breathing exercises, such as deep breathing, diaphragmatic breathing, and pursed-lip breathing, can help improve lung function, increase oxygenation, and reduce shortness of breath. These exercises can also help reduce anxiety and improve relaxation.

Pulmonary rehabilitation: Pulmonary rehabilitation is a comprehensive program that combines exercise, education, and support to help patients with lung disease improve their physical function and quality of life. Pulmonary rehabilitation programs may include aerobic and resistance exercises, breathing exercises, and education on disease management and lifestyle modifications.

Yoga and tai chi: Yoga and tai chi are gentle forms of exercise that incorporate stretching, breathing, and relaxation techniques. These practices can help improve flexibility, balance, and relaxation, as well as reduce stress and anxiety.

Massage therapy: Massage therapy is a hands-on approach that manipulates soft tissues in order to enhance circulation, ease muscle tension, and induce a state of relaxation. This form of therapy has been known to alleviate pain, fatigue, and anxiety, while also promoting better sleep quality and overall health and wellness.

It is important for lung cancer patients to work with a qualified healthcare professional, such as a physical therapist or exercise specialist, to develop an individualized exercise and physical therapy plan. The healthcare professional can evaluate the patient's physical function, medical history, and treatment plan, and design an appropriate exercise program that meets the patient's specific needs and goals.

How to incorporate exercise into daily routine

Lung cancer patients can incorporate exercise into their daily routine to improve their overall health, manage symptoms, and boost their recovery. However, it's crucial to consult with a healthcare professional before starting any exercise program to ensure it's safe and appropriate for your condition.

Here are some tips on how lung cancer patients can incorporate exercise into their daily routine:

Start slow and gradually increase intensity

It's essential to start slowly and gradually increase the intensity of your exercise routine. Begin with gentle exercises such as walking, stretching, or yoga, and then gradually increase the duration and intensity of your workouts over time. This helps you avoid fatigue, shortness of breath, and other side effects associated with lung cancer.

Choose low-impact exercises

Lung cancer patients should choose low-impact exercises such as swimming, cycling, or using an elliptical machine that puts less stress on their joints and lungs. These exercises can also help improve cardiovascular health, enhance lung function, and boost overall strength.

Incorporate resistance training

Resistance training is a great way to build muscle mass and improve bone density, which can be particularly beneficial for lung cancer patients who may experience muscle wasting due to chemotherapy and radiation therapy. Strength training exercises such as squats, lunges, and bicep curls can help improve balance, coordination, and overall physical function.

Use breathing techniques

Lung cancer patients can use breathing techniques such as pursed-lip breathing or diaphragmatic breathing to manage shortness of breath during exercise. These techniques can help increase lung capacity, reduce anxiety, and improve overall respiratory function.

Find a workout buddy or support group

Exercising with a workout buddy or joining a support group can provide motivation, accountability, and social support during your recovery. A supportive network can also help you stay positive and manage the emotional and psychological impact of a lung cancer diagnosis.

Schedule exercise into your daily routine

Scheduling exercise into your daily routine can help make it a regular habit. Choose a time of day when you have the most energy, and plan your workouts in advance. This can help you stay consistent and motivated.

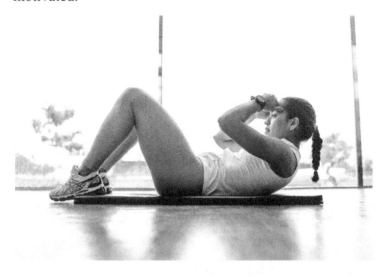

"When one door closes, another opens; but we often look so long and so regretfully upon the closed door that we do not see the one which has opened for us." - Alexander Graham Bell

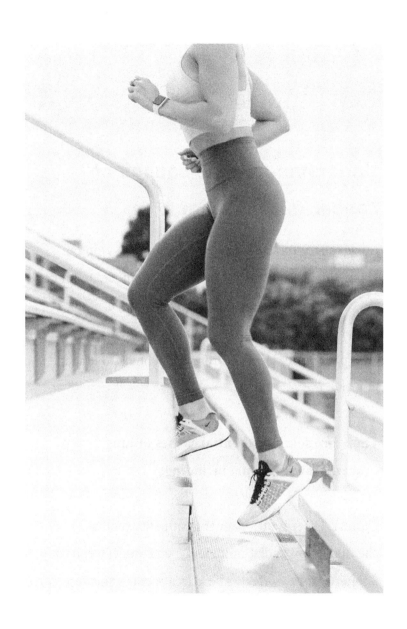

How to beat lung cancer 80

Chapter 6: Managing Fatigue and Sleep Issues

Understanding the causes of cancer-related fatigue

Lung cancer-related fatigue is a common symptom experienced by individuals with lung cancer, and it can have a significant impact on their quality of life. Understanding the causes of this fatigue is important for both patients and healthcare professionals to manage and improve it.

There are several potential causes of lung cancer-related fatigue, including:

Cancer Treatment: Cancer treatments such as chemotherapy, radiation therapy, and surgery can cause fatigue as a side effect. These treatments can cause damage to healthy cells and tissues in the body, leading to fatigue and other symptoms.

Cancer Progression: As lung cancer progresses, it can cause physical changes in the body that contribute to fatigue. Tumors can grow and spread, which can cause pain, difficulty breathing, and other symptoms that can make it harder for individuals to engage in their usual activities.

Anemia: Anemia is a common condition in individuals with lung cancer, and it can contribute to fatigue. Anemia occurs when the body doesn't have enough red blood cells to carry oxygen to the body's tissues, which can cause weakness, tiredness, and other symptoms.

Poor Nutrition: Poor nutrition can also contribute to fatigue in individuals with lung cancer. Cancer treatment can cause changes in appetite and digestion, and individuals may not be getting the nutrients they need to maintain their energy levels.

Depression and Anxiety: Depression and anxiety are common in individuals with cancer, and they can contribute to fatigue. These conditions can cause changes in sleep patterns, decrease motivation, and affect energy levels.

Lack of Physical Activity: Lack of physical activity can also contribute to fatigue. Individuals with lung cancer may have difficulty engaging in physical activity due to symptoms such as pain, shortness of breath, and fatigue. However, regular physical activity can help improve energy levels and reduce fatigue.

Managing lung cancer-related fatigue involves identifying the underlying causes and addressing them as appropriate. This may include adjusting cancer treatment to minimize side effects, treating anemia with medication, addressing poor nutrition with dietary changes or supplements, and addressing depression and anxiety with counseling or medication.

Coping strategies for managing fatigue

Lung cancer-related fatigue is a common and often debilitating symptom experienced by many patients with lung cancer. Coping strategies for managing lung cancer-related fatigue can help to alleviate symptoms and improve the overall quality of life. Here are some effective coping strategies for managing lung cancer-related fatigue:

Energy conservation: One of the most effective coping strategies for managing lung cancer-related fatigue is energy conservation. Patients should conserve energy by pacing themselves throughout the day, taking frequent rest breaks, and delegating tasks that require a lot of energy to others.

Exercise: Exercise has been shown to improve energy levels and reduce fatigue in lung cancer patients. Patients should consult with their healthcare provider before beginning an exercise program and start with gentle exercises such as walking or stretching.

Sleep: Getting enough sleep is essential for managing lung cancer-related fatigue. Patients should practice good sleep hygiene, such as sticking to a regular sleep schedule, avoiding caffeine and alcohol, and creating a comfortable sleep environment.

Nutrition: A balanced and healthy diet can help to improve energy levels and reduce fatigue. Patients should aim to eat a diet rich in fruits, vegetables, whole grains, and lean proteins.

Stress reduction: Stress can worsen fatigue symptoms, so it's essential to find ways to reduce stress. Patients can try relaxation techniques such as deep breathing, meditation, or yoga.

Support: Lung cancer patients can benefit greatly from support groups, counseling, or therapy. Talking with others who have experienced similar symptoms can provide a sense of comfort and understanding.

Medications: There are medications available that can help to manage fatigue symptoms, such as stimulants or antidepressants. Patients should discuss the use of medications with their healthcare provider.

Alternative therapies: There are alternative therapies available that may help alleviate fatigue symptoms, such as acupuncture, massage, and herbal supplements. However, it is important for patients to seek guidance from their healthcare provider before trying any of these complementary or alternative therapies.

Sleep issues and how to improve sleep quality

Sleep issues are common among lung cancer patients due to various factors such as pain, anxiety, medication side effects, and physical discomfort. These sleep issues can have a negative impact on a patient's quality of life, as sleep plays a crucial role in the body's overall health and well-being. However, there are several strategies that can help improve sleep quality for lung cancer patients.

Establish a regular sleep routine
Individuals diagnosed with lung cancer should strive to maintain a consistent sleep schedule by going to bed and waking up at the same time daily, even on weekends. This promotes the regulation of the body's internal clock, enhancing the ability to fall asleep at night and awaken in the morning.

Create a relaxing sleep environment

Creating a relaxing sleep environment can help lung cancer patients fall asleep faster and stay asleep longer. This includes keeping the bedroom cool, quiet, and dark, and removing any distractions such as televisions or electronic devices.

Practice relaxation techniques

Relaxation techniques such as deep breathing, progressive muscle relaxation, and meditation can help reduce stress and anxiety, making it easier for lung cancer patients to fall asleep.

Exercise regularly

Regular exercise can help lung cancer patients feel more relaxed and reduce stress, which can improve sleep quality. However, it is important to avoid vigorous exercise close to bedtime, as this can have the opposite effect and make it harder to fall asleep.

Avoid caffeine and alcohol

The consumption of caffeine and alcohol can interfere with the natural sleep cycle and impede the ability to initiate sleep. If you are a lung cancer patient, it is advisable to refrain from consuming these substances, particularly during the night.

Manage pain and discomfort

Pain and discomfort are common among lung cancer patients, and can make it difficult to get comfortable and fall asleep. Working with a healthcare provider to manage pain and discomfort can help improve sleep quality.

Consult with a healthcare provider

Lung cancer patients should consult with their healthcare provider if they are experiencing sleep issues, as there may be underlying medical conditions or medication side effects that are contributing to the problem. The healthcare provider may also recommend medications or other treatments to help improve sleep quality.

"Don't count the days, make the days count." - Muhammad Ali

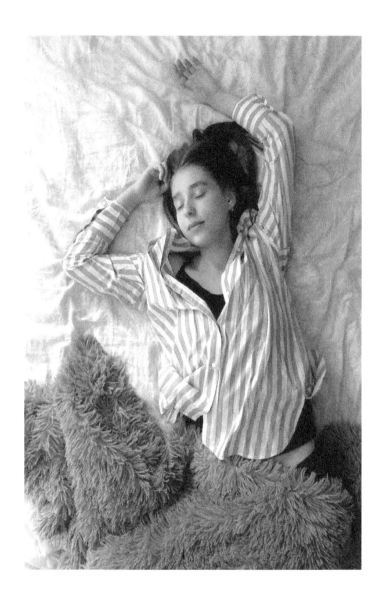

Chapter 7: Support and Resources for Lung Cancer Patients

Importance of support during recovery

The journey of recovery from lung cancer can be challenging and often requires extensive medical treatment and support from family, friends, and healthcare professionals. Adequate support during recovery is crucial to help lung cancer patients manage their symptoms, cope with emotional distress, and improve their overall quality of life.

Here are some of the key reasons why support is essential during recovery for lung cancer patients:

Coping with physical symptoms: Lung cancer treatment can cause physical side effects such as fatigue, nausea, pain, and shortness of breath. Support from healthcare professionals can help patients manage these symptoms by providing medications, therapies, and advice on self-care practices.

Managing emotional distress: A cancer diagnosis can be emotionally distressing, and patients may experience anxiety, depression, and fear. Support from family and friends can provide emotional comfort and reassurance, while counseling and therapy can help patients learn coping strategies to manage their emotions.

Navigating the healthcare system: Managing medical appointments, insurance, and treatment plans can be overwhelming for lung cancer patients. Support from healthcare professionals and caregivers can help patients navigate the healthcare system and ensure that they receive timely and appropriate treatment.

Improving the quality of life: Support from loved ones and healthcare professionals can improve the patient's overall quality of life. Social support can provide a sense of belonging and reduce feelings of isolation, while medical support can improve physical health and increase the patient's ability to perform daily activities.

Enhancing recovery outcomes: Studies have shown that support during recovery can enhance the patient's recovery outcomes. Patients who have a strong support system are more likely to adhere to treatment plans, experience fewer complications, and have better long-term survival rates.

Types of support and resources available for lung cancer patients

Coping with lung cancer can be a challenging experience, and patients require support and resources to help them manage their diagnosis, treatment, and recovery. In this part, we will discuss the different types of support and resources available for lung cancer patients.

Medical Support:
Access to medical assistance is crucial for individuals with lung cancer, encompassing the diagnosis, treatment, and ongoing monitoring provided by healthcare experts

like oncologists, pulmonologists, and other specialists. Surgery, radiation therapy, chemotherapy, and targeted therapy are among the treatment choices for lung cancer. A collaborative team approach is commonly employed to ensure that patients with lung cancer receive comprehensive care.

Emotional Support:

Cancer diagnosis and treatment can be emotionally challenging for patients and their families. Emotional support can come in many forms, such as support groups, counseling, and therapy. Support groups bring together people who are experiencing similar challenges and provide a space for them to share their experiences, offer support, and learn from one another. Counseling and therapy provide patients and their families with a safe and confidential space to express their thoughts and feelings and learn coping strategies to manage the emotional impact of cancer.

Financial Support:

Cancer treatment can be expensive, and patients may need financial support to manage the costs associated with their treatment. Some organizations offer financial assistance to help with the cost of treatment, such as co-pay assistance and transportation costs. Patients may also be eligible for government-sponsored programs such as Medicare and Medicaid.

Educational Support:

Educational support is important for patients with lung cancer to understand their diagnosis, treatment options, and self-care. Educational resources can come in many forms, such as brochures, videos, and websites. Some organizations provide education and resources specific to lung cancer, such as the American Lung Association and the Lung Cancer Research Foundation.

Practical Support:

Practical support can help lung cancer patients with everyday activities, such as transportation to and from appointments, meals, and housekeeping. Some organizations offer volunteer services that provide practical support to cancer patients and their families.

Spiritual Support:

For some patients, spiritual support can help them cope with cancer. Spiritual support can come in many forms, such as chaplaincy services and pastoral care. Some hospitals and cancer centers offer spiritual support services to patients and their families.

Finding and connecting with support groups

A diagnosis of lung cancer can be a daunting and challenging experience for patients and their loved ones. It can be emotionally and physically overwhelming, and support groups can help cope with the disease. Support groups provide a safe space where people can share their experiences, feelings, and concerns, and connect with others who are going through a similar journey. In this section, we will discuss how to find and connect with support groups for lung cancer patients.

Reach out to your medical team: Your medical team can provide you with information on support groups for lung cancer patients. They may have a list of local or online support groups that they can recommend. They may also be able to refer you to a social worker who can help you find support.

Online resources: The internet can be a useful tool to find support groups. There are various online forums and communities for lung cancer patients where you can connect with others who have been through a similar experience. Websites such as Cancer Support Community, American Cancer Society, and Lung Cancer Alliance provide information on support groups, including online communities.

Social media: Social media platforms such as Facebook and Twitter have groups and communities that offer support for lung cancer patients. You can search for groups using keywords such as "lung cancer support" or "lung cancer patients" and join the groups that appeal to you.

National organizations: National organizations such as the American Lung Association and the Lung Cancer Research Foundation offer support groups for lung cancer patients. These organizations have local chapters and offer online support groups as well. They also provide educational resources and other services.

Local cancer centers: Cancer centers often have support groups for their patients, and they can be a great resource for finding support groups in your area. You can contact your local cancer center or hospital and ask if they offer support groups for lung cancer patients.

Word of mouth: Word of mouth can be a powerful tool in finding support groups. Talk to your friends and family, and ask if they know of any support groups for lung cancer patients. They may have personal experience or know someone who has gone through a similar experience.

For individuals with lung cancer, reaching out to a support group can serve as a crucial source of support.

By doing so, they can alleviate any sentiments of isolation and foster a sense of belonging within a community. Identifying a support group that can cater to their specific needs and offers the desired type of assistance is imperative. It may require attending several groups before finding the ideal fit. Remember that there are people who are willing to extend their help and support, and you are not alone in this journey.

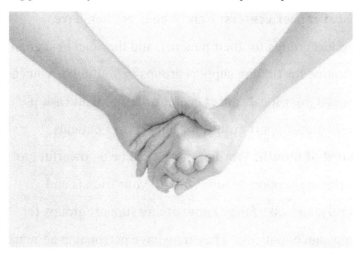

"You have within you right now, everything you need to deal with whatever the world can throw at you." - Brian Tracy

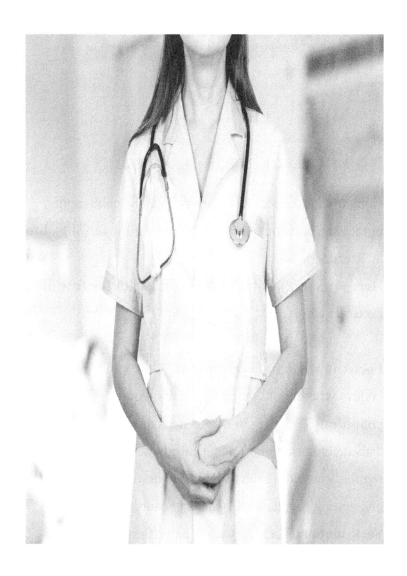

Chapter 8: Life After Lung Cancer

Coping with the fear of recurrence

Coping with the fear of recurrence can be challenging, but it is an essential part of living a healthy, fulfilling life after cancer.

Here are some strategies for coping with the fear of recurrence:

Focus on what you can control: While you cannot control whether or not cancer recurs, you can control your lifestyle choices and take steps to reduce your risk. This includes maintaining a healthy diet, exercising regularly, avoiding tobacco and excessive alcohol use, and getting regular check-ups and cancer screenings.

Seek support: Talking with friends, family, or a therapist can help you process your emotions and fears. Consider joining a support group for cancer survivors or connecting with online communities where you can share your experiences and learn from others.

Practice mindfulness: Mindfulness techniques, such as deep breathing, meditation, and yoga, can help you manage anxiety and reduce stress. These practices can also help you stay present at the moment and appreciate the good things in life.

Educate yourself: Understanding the signs and symptoms of cancer recurrence can help you be proactive about your health. Work with your healthcare team to create a plan for monitoring and detecting any changes in your health.

Take care of your mental and emotional health: Cancer can take a toll on your mental and emotional well-being, and it's essential to prioritize self-care. Consider seeking counseling or therapy, practicing relaxation techniques, or engaging in activities that bring you joy and relaxation.

Find ways to stay positive: Cancer survivors often report a newfound appreciation for life and a desire to live more fully. Focus on the positive things in your life, such as spending time with loved ones, pursuing your passions, and setting goals for the future.

Physical and emotional changes after lung cancer treatment

Lung cancer is a serious medical condition that can cause significant physical and emotional changes in a person's life. Treatment for lung cancer, such as surgery, chemotherapy, radiation therapy, or a combination of these, can also have a profound impact on a patient's body and mind. In this article, we will explore the physical and emotional changes that may occur after lung cancer treatment.

Physical changes after lung cancer treatment:
Fatigue: Fatigue is a common side effect of lung cancer treatment. Patients may experience extreme tiredness, weakness, and lack of energy for several weeks or months after their treatment. This can be due to the side

effects of chemotherapy, radiation, or surgery, and it may take time to recover.

Shortness of breath: Depending on the extent of lung cancer and the type of treatment, patients may experience shortness of breath after their treatment. This can be due to damage to the lungs, decreased lung function, or scarring from surgery or radiation therapy.

Changes in appetite: Patients may experience changes in their appetite after lung cancer treatment. Some may have a decreased appetite, while others may experience an increased appetite due to the side effects of treatment.

Weight loss: Weight loss is common among lung cancer patients due to a decrease in appetite and changes in metabolism. Patients may lose muscle mass, which can lead to weakness and fatigue.

Hair loss: Chemotherapy can cause hair loss, including the loss of eyebrows and eyelashes.

Pain: Pain is common after surgery, especially in the chest area. Patients may also experience pain due to radiation therapy, nerve damage, or scar tissue.

Lymphedema: Lymphedema is a condition in which excess fluid builds up in the arms or legs, causing swelling. This can occur after surgery or radiation therapy that involves the lymph nodes.

Emotional changes after lung cancer treatment:

Anxiety and depression: Lung cancer treatment can be stressful, and patients may experience anxiety and depression. This can be due to fear of recurrence, changes in body image, and concerns about the future.

Fear of recurrence: After lung cancer treatment, patients may worry about cancer coming back. This fear can be overwhelming and may cause anxiety.

Changes in body image: Surgery, radiation therapy, and chemotherapy can cause changes in body image, such as scarring, hair loss, and weight changes. These changes can affect a patient's self-esteem and confidence.

Post-traumatic stress disorder (PTSD): Some patients may develop PTSD after lung cancer treatment, especially if they had a traumatic experience during their treatment.

Relationship changes: Lung cancer treatment can affect relationships with family, friends, and romantic partners.

Patients may feel isolated, and their loved ones may struggle to understand what they are going through.

Financial stress: Lung cancer treatment can be expensive, and patients may experience financial stress. This can be due to medical bills, time off work, and other expenses associated with treatment.

Moving forward with a new perspective on life

The first step to moving forward with a new perspective on life for lung cancer patients is to acknowledge the diagnosis and the emotions that come with it. It's essential to give yourself time to process and come to terms with the diagnosis. It's also important to understand that lung cancer is a treatable disease, and there are many treatment options available that can improve your prognosis.

The next step is to build a support system. This can include family, friends, and healthcare professionals.

Support groups can also be a great resource for patients and their loved ones to connect with others who are going through similar experiences. Talking with others who have been through a similar journey can provide valuable insight, comfort, and encouragement.

Taking care of your physical health is also important when moving forward with a new perspective on life after a lung cancer diagnosis. It's essential to maintain a healthy lifestyle by eating a balanced diet, exercising regularly, and getting enough rest. Quitting smoking is also critical for patients with lung cancer, as it can improve treatment outcomes and reduce the risk of cancer recurrence.

Another crucial aspect of moving forward with a new perspective on life for lung cancer patients is to focus on positivity and mindfulness. This can include practicing meditation, yoga, or other relaxation techniques to reduce stress and anxiety. It's also important to celebrate small victories and take things one day at a time. This can help patients stay positive and focused on their treatment and recovery.

Lastly, it's essential to stay informed and involved in your treatment plan. Ask questions, research treatment options, and discuss any concerns or side effects with your healthcare team. Being an active participant in your treatment can help you feel more in control and give you a sense of purpose and direction.

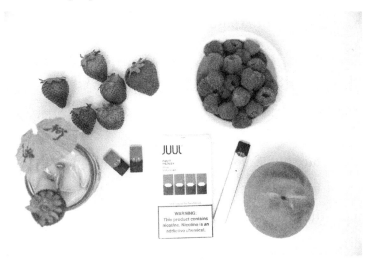

"Every moment is a fresh beginning." - T.S. Eliot

Chapter 9: Preventing Lung Cancer

Tips to Minimize the Chance of Developing Lung Cancer

Lung cancer is a type of cancer that develops in the tissues of the lungs, most often in people who smoke or have a history of exposure to carcinogens. However, there are several strategies that can help reduce the risk of developing lung cancer. Here are some of the most successful methods:

Quit smoking: Smoking is the most significant risk factor for lung cancer, and quitting smoking is the single most effective way to reduce the risk of developing this disease. According to the American Cancer Society, smokers who quit before the age of 50 can cut their risk of dying from lung cancer by 50%.

Avoid secondhand smoke: Secondhand smoke is also a significant risk factor for lung cancer. Therefore, it is essential to avoid exposure to smoke from other people's cigarettes or other tobacco products.

Limit exposure to carcinogens: Exposure to certain carcinogens, such as radon, asbestos, and air pollution, can increase the risk of developing lung cancer. Therefore, it is important to take steps to limit exposure to these substances. For example, testing for radon in homes and workplaces and installing ventilation systems can help reduce exposure to this harmful gas.

Eat a healthy diet: A diet rich in fruits and vegetables, whole grains, and lean protein sources can help reduce the risk of developing lung cancer. Foods high in antioxidants, such as berries, tomatoes, and leafy greens, are especially beneficial.

Exercise regularly: Regular exercise can help maintain a healthy weight, boost the immune system, and reduce inflammation in the body, all of which can help reduce the risk of developing lung cancer.

Get regular check-ups: Regular check-ups with a healthcare provider can help detect lung cancer in its early stages when it is most treatable. People at high risk of developing lung cancer, such as current or former smokers, may need to undergo regular screening tests, such as a low-dose CT scan.

Consider genetic testing: Some people may have a higher risk of developing lung cancer due to genetic factors. Genetic testing can help identify individuals who are at increased risk, allowing for earlier detection and more effective treatment.

Screening and early detection

Early detection and screening of lung cancer can significantly improve survival rates and reduce mortality. This is because lung cancer often does not cause any noticeable symptoms in its early stages, and by the time symptoms do appear, the cancer has often progressed to a more advanced stage.

Screening for lung cancer involves testing individuals who are at high risk for developing the disease but do not have any symptoms. The goal of screening is to detect lung cancer at an early stage when it is more treatable. Currently, the most common screening method for lung cancer is low-dose computed tomography (CT) scanning.

The National Lung Screening Trial (NLST) conducted in the United States found that screening high-risk individuals with low-dose CT scanning reduced lung cancer mortality by 20% compared to screening with chest X-rays. The NLST recommended screening individuals who meet the following criteria:

Aged 55 to 80 years
Have a smoking history of at least 30 pack-years (i.e., smoked one pack per day for 30 years or two packs per day for 15 years)
Currently smoking or have quit within the past 15 years
However, it is important to note that screening with CT scanning can also have risks, such as exposure to radiation and false-positive results that may lead to unnecessary invasive procedures.

It's crucial to emphasize that using screening methods alone should not be considered a replacement for quitting smoking. Quitting smoking is still the most efficient method of preventing lung cancer.

In addition to screening, early detection of lung cancer can also be achieved through awareness and recognizing the signs and symptoms of the disease. These may include:

A persistent cough that does not go away or worsens over time
Shortness of breath
Chest pain
Hoarseness
Fatigue
Unexplained weight loss
Coughing up blood
If an individual experiences any of these symptoms, they should consult their healthcare provider for evaluation.

Importance of quitting smoking

Smoking is one of the leading causes of lung cancer, and quitting smoking is of utmost importance for lung cancer patients. Lung cancer is a type of cancer that affects the lungs and is usually caused by smoking. According to the American Cancer Society, smoking is responsible for 80% of lung cancer cases. Lung cancer patients who continue to smoke after their diagnosis have a higher risk of mortality than those who quit smoking. In this article, we will discuss the importance of quitting smoking for lung cancer patients.

Improve Treatment Outcomes

Quitting smoking is essential for lung cancer patients because it can improve their treatment outcomes. Smoking can reduce the effectiveness of cancer treatments such as radiation therapy, chemotherapy, and surgery. Smoking can also increase the risk of complications during and after treatment. By quitting smoking, patients can improve their overall health, increase their chances of responding to treatment, and decrease their risk of complications.

Reduce the Risk of Cancer Recurrence

Lung cancer patients who continue to smoke after their diagnosis have a higher risk of cancer recurrence than those who quit smoking. Smoking can promote the growth and spread of cancer cells in the body, making it more difficult to treat cancer. By quitting smoking, patients can reduce the risk of cancer recurrence and improve their chances of surviving the disease.

Improve Lung Function

The act of smoking has the potential to harm the lungs and impair their overall functioning. Lung cancer patients who smoke may have a harder time breathing, and their lung function may be compromised. By quitting smoking, patients can improve their lung function and make it easier to breathe. This can improve their quality of life and help them better tolerate cancer treatments.

Reduce the Risk of Second Cancer

Lung cancer patients who smoke are at an increased risk of developing second cancer. This is because smoking can damage the DNA in cells, leading to the development of cancer. By quitting smoking, patients can reduce their risk of developing second cancer, which can improve their overall health and quality of life.

Improve Overall Health

Quitting smoking can improve lung cancer patient's overall health and quality of life. Smoking can cause a variety of health problems, including heart disease, stroke, and respiratory infections. By quitting smoking, patients can reduce their risk of developing these health problems and improve their overall health.

"Courage doesn't always roar. Sometimes courage is the quiet voice at the end of the day saying, 'I will try again tomorrow.'" - Mary Anne Radmacher

Bonus: 30 nutritional dense food for lung cancer patients

Here are 20 nutrient-dense foods that may be beneficial for lung cancer patients:

Broccoli: Contains compounds that may help prevent lung cancer and boost the immune system.

Spinach: Rich in antioxidants and vitamin C, which may help reduce inflammation and protect against cancer.

Carrots: High in beta-carotene, which may help reduce the risk of lung cancer and improve lung function.

Tomatoes: Contains lycopene, which may help prevent lung cancer and reduce inflammation.

Garlic: May help boost the immune system and reduce the risk of lung cancer.

Onions: Rich in quercetin, which has anti-inflammatory and antioxidant properties.

Blueberries: Contains antioxidants that may help protect against cancer and boost the immune system.

Avocado: Contains healthy fats and vitamin E, which may help reduce inflammation and improve lung function.

Walnuts: Rich in omega-3 fatty acids, which may help reduce inflammation and improve lung function.

Salmon: Contains omega-3 fatty acids, which may help reduce inflammation and improve lung function.

Sweet potatoes: High in vitamin A and antioxidants, which may help reduce the risk of lung cancer and boost the immune system.

Lentils: Rich in fiber and protein, which may help reduce inflammation and improve lung function.

Brazil nuts: Rich in selenium, which may help reduce the risk of lung cancer and improve lung function.

Green tea: Contains antioxidants and may help reduce the risk of lung cancer and improve lung function.

Turmeric: Contains curcumin, which has anti-inflammatory and antioxidant properties.

Citrus fruits: High in vitamin C, which may help reduce inflammation and boost the immune system.

Red bell peppers: Rich in vitamin C and antioxidants, which may help reduce inflammation and protect against cancer.

Dark chocolate: Contains flavonoids, which have anti-inflammatory and antioxidant properties.

Ginger: May help reduce inflammation and boost the immune system.

Mushrooms: Contains polysaccharides, which may help boost the immune system and reduce the risk of lung cancer.

Chia seeds: Rich in omega-3 fatty acids, fiber, and protein, which may help reduce inflammation and improve lung function.

Quinoa: A good source of fiber and protein, which may help reduce inflammation and improve lung function.

Pomegranates: Rich in antioxidants, which may help reduce inflammation and protect against cancer.

Cabbage: Contains compounds that may help prevent lung cancer and boost the immune system.

Almonds: Rich in healthy fats and vitamin E, which may help reduce inflammation and improve lung function.

Oats: Rich in fiber, which may help reduce inflammation and improve lung function.

Black beans: A good source of fiber and protein, which may help reduce inflammation and improve lung function.

Kiwi: Rich in vitamin C and antioxidants, which may help reduce inflammation and protect against cancer.

Pumpkin: Contains beta-carotene, which may help reduce the risk of lung cancer and improve lung function.

Green leafy vegetables (e.g., kale, collard greens, mustard greens): Rich in antioxidants and vitamin C, which may help reduce inflammation and protect against cancer.

It's important to note that while certain foods may have potential benefits for lung cancer patients, it's always best to consult with a healthcare provider and a registered dietitian to develop an individualized nutrition plan.

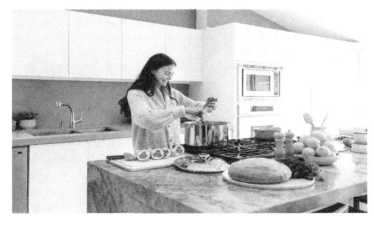